Chemo Cookbook

Healthy & Delicious Recipes to Enjoy During Chemo Therapy

BY

Daniel Humphreys

Copyright 2019 Daniel Humphreys

License Notes

No part of this Book can be reproduced in any form or by any means including print, electronic, scanning or photocopying unless prior permission is granted by the author.

All ideas, suggestions and guidelines mentioned here are written for informative purposes. While the author has taken every possible step to ensure accuracy, all readers are advised to follow information at their own risk. The author cannot be held responsible for personal and/or commercial damages in case of misinterpreting and misunderstanding any part of this Book

Table of Contents

Introduction

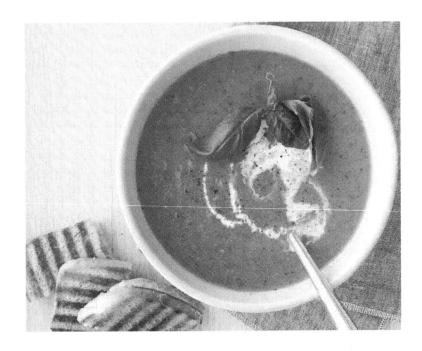

Did you recently start Chemo Therapy treatments? Have you released that food has begun to become more, and more, tasteless with each time that you eat? No, you aren't going crazy, and no, you are not losing you excellent cooking skills. The culprit for this is actually the radiation that you are now being subjected to in your treatments. The extensive exposure to the radiation as slowly been affecting your taste buds, and will, unfortunately, continue to affect them throughout the term of your treatment.

So, what can you do to combat this? All you can do right now is focus on consuming nourishing foods that your body will be able to tolerate without that pesky side that you may already begin to experience like a sore throat, weight loss, neutropenia, and nausea. Luckily in this Chemo Therapy Cookbook, we will be exploring 30 simple, healthy and delicious recipes that you will kickstart your taste buds, and have you falling in love with food all over again. Best of all, the fun begins right now! Let's dive right in.

Chicken and White Bean Soup

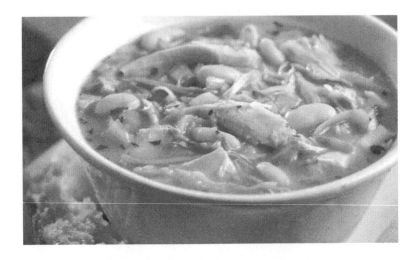

We all know chicken soup is great for the common flu, but did you know that it's soothing, protein packed goodness is also great for chemo patients? Here's one such recipe that uses extremely flavorful with, and easy to digest.

Serving Size: 6

Overall Time: 40 Minutes

Ingredients:

- Rotisserie chicken (3 cups, chopped)
- Chicken Broth (6 cups, low sodium)
- Water (2 cups)
- White Beans (15oz., canned, rinsed)
- Oil (1 tbsp.)
- Celery (2 stalks, chopped)
- Carrots (3, peeled, chopped)
- Onion (1, diced)
- Salt and pepper (1 tsp. each)

Directions:

1. Remove the skin and bones from rotisserie chicken and shred.

2. Add the celery, carrots, and onion and sauté in 1 tbsp. of oil over a low to medium flame until the onions are glassy (roughly 10 mins).

3. Pour in chicken broth and simmer for a further 10 mins.

4. Add the chicken and the beans; allow to cook for five minutes.

5. Season to taste and serve.

Lemon, Broccoli and Garlic Penne Pasta

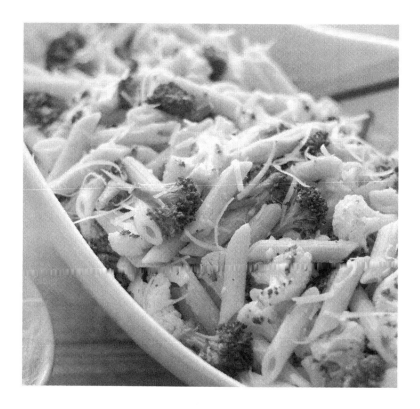

Pasta is usually very filling and quite easy to digest, perfect if you need to build up your weight after treatment.

Serving Size: 4

Overall Time: 35 Minutes

Ingredients:

- pasta (½ lb.)
- broccoli (5 cups)
- olive oil (1/4 cup)
- garlic (10 cloves, thinly sliced)
- chicken broth (1/2 cup, low sodium)
- Zest of one lemon, grated
- parmesan cheese (1/4 cup, grated)
- salt and pepper (1/4 tsp., to taste)

Directions:

1. Cook pasta following manufacturer's instructions on the packet; add broccoli three minutes before cooking is completed. When cooked, drain and put aside.

2. In a suitable size skillet, heat olive oil over medium heat. Add garlic slices and sauté for 2 mins. until color appears.

3. Pour in the broth and allow it to boil; reduce flame and simmer until the liquid has evaporated to about half of the regular amount. Stir constantly to prevent the garlic from sticking to the pan.

4. Add the pasta, zest of lemon and the broccoli; stir until heated through.

5. Season with salt and pepper and top with grated parmesan cheese. Serve.

Chili Con Carne

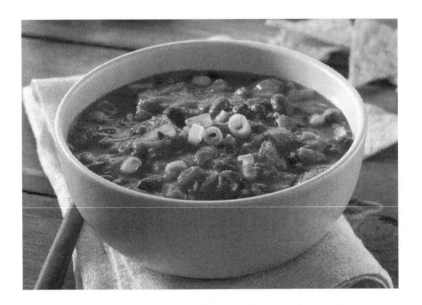

When you are in a hurry or short on energy, one-pot meals are always a great idea. Chili Con Carne can be made as mild or as spicy as desired. Can be accompanied with plain rice and can be frozen for future dinners.

Serving Size: 4

Overall Time: 50 Minutes

Ingredients:

- lean ground beef (1/2 lb.)
- oil (1 tbsp)
- onion (1, diced)
- garlic (1 clove)
- chopped tomatoes (1, 14 oz can)
- tomato paste (3 oz.)
- mushrooms (1 cup)
- bell pepper (1 red, sliced)
- chili powder (1/2 tsp.)
- ground cumin (1/2 tsp.)
- ground cilantro (1/2 tsp.)
- kidney beans (1, 14 oz. can drain)
- chili pepper (1, chopped; optional)
- salt and pepper (1/4 tsp. each, to taste)

Directions:

1. Over medium heat, sauté onions and garlic in a saucepan until they are translucent.

2. Stir in ground beef until it is golden brown (about four to five minutes). Add spices and the chili (if being used) and mix until all are combined.

3. Add the canned tomatoes and tomato paste, lower flame and simmer for roughly 12 to 15 minutes.

4. Add kidney beans, bell peppers, and mushrooms; cook for a further 10 minutes. Serve as desired.

Winter Veggie Pita Pizza

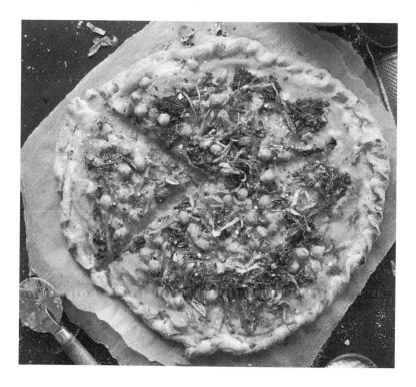

Of course, you can make a healthy, tasty pizza! This is a great choice for a nutritious light lunch or dinner with a nice salad.

Serving Size: 4

Overall Time: 40 Minutes

Ingredients:

- pita bread (4 whole-wheat)
- extra-virgin olive oil (2 tsp.)
- butternut squash (1 cup, cubed)
- brussels sprouts (1 cup, quartered)
- red onion (1/2 cup, sliced)
- ricotta cheese (1/2 cup, part-skim)
- pecans (2 tbsp., chopped)
- fresh sage (1 tbsp., chopped)
- parmesan cheese (8 tsp., grated)
- cinnamon (1/4 tsp.)

Directions:

1. Heat oven to 425 degrees F. Place oil in a medium bowl along with brussels sprouts and butternut squash and toss until combined.

2. Sprinkle with cinnamon; transfer vegetables to a baking sheet and bake in preheated oven for 20 minutes, turning vegetables halfway through.

3. When vegetables have completed cooking, spread the ricotta cheese on each pita bread.

4. On baking tray arrange pita bread on a tray, and place all other ingredients evenly around bread then sprinkle parmesan cheese on top of each.

5. Place directly on a rack in the oven and bake for 7 mins. or until pita bread is crispy and cheese melted.

Prawn Risotto

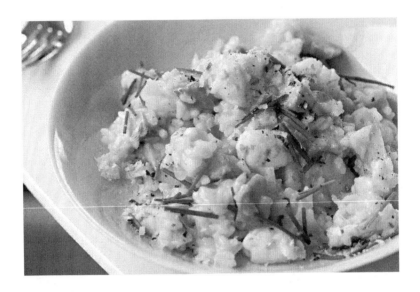

Prawns are not only delicious, but they are also a great source of omega-3 and protein. They are slightly high in cholesterol, however, so beware of the amount you consume if you were advised by your doctor to watch your cholesterol intake.

Serving Size: 4

Overall Time: 35 Minutes

Ingredients:

- olive oil (1 tbsp.)
- Arborio risotto rice (2 cups)
- Prawns (20 large)
- Green onions (1 cup, chopped)
- Garlic (4 cloves, minced)
- Fish broth (5 cups, low - sodium)
- Lemon juice (1/2 of a lemon)
- Parmesan cheese (1 tbsp.)
- Chives (1 tbsp., chopped)
- Salt and pepper (1/4 tsp., each, to taste)

Directions:

1. Set a skillet with oil over medium heat, and allow to get hot. Add garlic and green onions then cook, while stirring until soft.

2. Once soft, add vegetables, and rice, then allow the rice to toast slightly (about 2 minutes, while stirring).

3. Slowly add your broth, adding a little at a time, and stirring until almost fully absorbed. Repeat until rice is cooked (about 30 minutes).

4. While cooking rice, set your prawns to broil until cooked (about 5 minutes on high) then coarsely chop. Add to risotto and stir to evenly combine.

5. Add in your remaining ingredients, season with salt and pepper then serve.

Thai Chicken and Coconut Soup

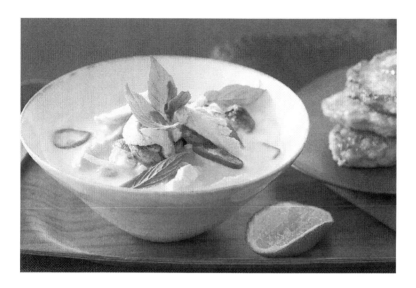

This delicious soup is nutrient dense, and the perfect addition to any day.

Serving Size: 4

Overall Time: 45 Minutes

Ingredients:

- Coconut oil (1 tbsp.)
- Chicken breast (½ lb., cubed)
- Onion (1 medium, chopped)
- Garlic (1 clove, minced)
- Ginger (1 tbsp., minced)
- Carrots (1 cup, diced)
- Chili Paste (½ tsp, roasted)
- Shiitake mushrooms (1 cup, sliced)
- Chicken stock (3 cups, low-sodium)
- Lime (1, zested, juiced)
- Fish sauce (1 tbsp.)
- Coconut milk (1 14oz can)
- Cilantro (¼ cup, chopped)

Directions:

1. Set a large saucepan with oil on over medium heat, and allow to get hot.

2. Add chicken, and allow to brown on all sides. Set aside.

3. Add chili paste, garlic, ginger, onions, and carrots then cook, while stirring, until soft.

4. Add in your remaining ingredients, reduce heat, and allow to simmer for another 5 minutes. Serve.

Herby Chicken Breasts

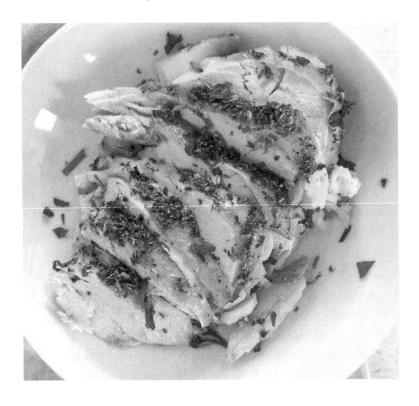

Enjoy this delicious chicken with your favorite side, and rest assured that it will be easily digested.

Serving Size: 4

Overall Time: 20 Minutes

Ingredients:

- Chicken breasts (2, skinless, boneless, halved)
- Sesame oil (2 tsp.)
- Onion (½, diced)
- Ginger (½-inch, minced)
- Lime zest (½ tsp., grated)
- Cilantro (1 cup, chopped)
- Spearmint (1 cup)
- Olive oil (3 tbsp., extra virgin)
- Salt (½ tsp.)
- Pepper (1/4 tsp.)

Directions:

1. Add your salt, ginger, onion, pepper, sesame oil, lime zest, cilantro and spearmint to a food processor, and process until it forms a rough paste.

2. Use a mallet to flatten each chicken breast, spread half your marinade evenly over all your chicken pieces, flip then spread the other half evenly on the other side.

3. Set a skillet with oil over medium heat, and allow to get hot. Add your chicken pieces one at a time, and fry until cooked through (about 10 minutes, flipping half way through). Serve, and enjoy.

Old-Fashioned Chicken Noodle Soup

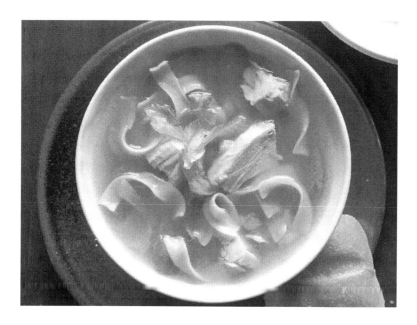

There's nothing better than a good bowl of old fashioned chicken soup. Here is an easy recipe that you can follow.

Serving Size: 4

Overall Time: 1 Hour 1 Minute

Ingredients:

- Chicken Stock (8 cups, fat-free, low-sodium)
- Chicken thighs (8 oz., skinless, boneless)
- Chicken breast (12 oz., skinless, boneless, halved)
- Carrots (2 cups, sliced diagonally)
- Celery (2 cups, sliced diagonally)
- Onion (1 cup, chopped)
- Egg noodles (6 oz.)
- Salt (1/2 tsp.)
- Black pepper (1/2 tsp.)

Directions:

1. Set a Dutch oven over medium heat with your first 3 ingredients and allow to come to a boil.

2. Once boiling, reduce heat to low then continue to simmer for about 20 minutes.

3. Set chicken aside, and allow to stand uncovered for 10 minutes. Chop into bite sized pieces, and set aside.

4. Add vegetables, cover, and allow to continue to simmer until fork tender (about 10 minutes) then add noodles, then allow to simmer until fork tender (about 6 minutes).

5. Add in your remaining ingredients, and continue to cook until chicken has been fully heated through. Season to taste and serve.

Cold Chicken Rice Salad

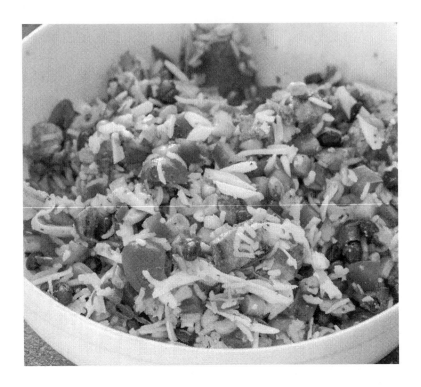

This salad is perfect for a hot day. Serve with fresh fruit, and enjoy all the nutrients in a delicious way.

Serving Size: 4

Overall Time: 1 Hour 10 Minutes

Ingredients:

- Chicken breast (12 oz., skinless, boneless, halved)
- Salt (3/4 tsp.)
- Black pepper (3/4 tsp.)
- Cooking spray
- Rice (3/4 cup, uncooked)
- Lemon juice (3 tbsp.)
- Olive oil (2 tbsp.)
- Cranberries (1/3 cup, dried)
- Celery (1/4 cup, diced)
- Green onion (1/4 cup, thinly sliced)
- Red bell pepper (1/4 cup, diced
- Olives (1/4 cup, chopped, pimiento-stuffed)
- Lettuce leaves (12, green leaf, torn)
- Lemon wedges (2)

Directions:

1. Set your oven to preheat 400 degrees F, and season your chicken with half your salt, and pepper.

2. Set a lightly greased skillet over medium heat, and allow to get hot.

3. Add chicken, and cook for about 3 minutes, flip then transfer the skillet to your oven.

4. Allow to bake until fully cooked (about 8 minutes).

5. Remove from heat, and allow to let stand for about 5 minutes.

6. Allow to chill in the refrigerator until cool. Shred, and serve.

Lemon Risotto with Peas, Tarragon, and Leeks

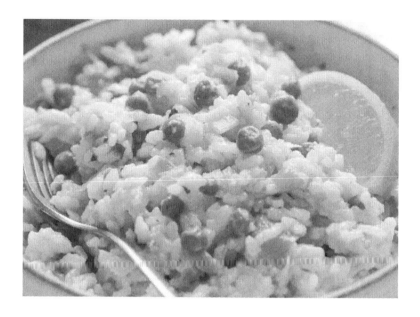

This recipe is simple to make but bold in flavor.

Serving Size: 8

Overall Time: 40 Minutes

Ingredients:

- Green Peas (1 cup, fresh, blanched)
- Chicken stock (4 cups, warm)
- Olive oil (2 tbsp., extra-virgin)
- Leek (1 1/2 cups, finely chopped)
- Shallots (1/2 cup, chopped)
- Arborio rice (1 cup, uncooked)
- White wine (3 tbsp., dry)
- Parmesan cheese (1/2 cup, grated)
- Lemon rind (1 tsp., grated)
- Lemon juice (2 tbsp.)
- Salt (1/2 tsp.)
- Black pepper (1/8 tsp.)
- Tarragon (2 tbsp., chopped)
- Butter (1 tbsp.)

Directions:

1. Set a skillet with butter over medium heat, and allow to get hot. Add shallots, and leeks then cook, while stirring until soft.

2. Once soft, add rice then allow the rice to toast slightly (about 2 minutes, while stirring). Add your wine, and allow to cook for 30 seconds.

3. Slowly add your broth, adding a little at a time, and stirring until almost fully absorbed. Repeat until rice is cooked (about 30 minutes).

4. Add in your remaining ingredients, season with salt and pepper then serve.

Rice Pudding

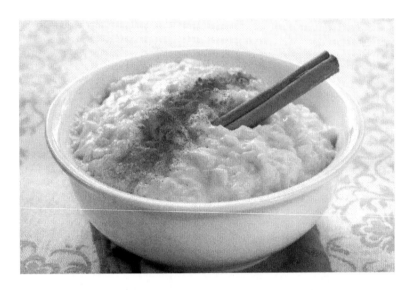

If you are a dessert lover, there's no need to give that up. Instead, enjoy healthier alternatives such as this delicious rice pudding.

Serving Size: 12

Overall Time: 1 Hour 30 Minutes

Ingredients:

- Milk (8 cups, 2%)
- Sugar (1 cup)
- Butter (2 tbsp.)
- Rice (1 1/2 cups, long-grain)
- Salt (1/4 tsp.)
- Egg (1 large)
- Raisins (1/2 cup, golden)
- Amaretto (1/4 cup, almond)
- Vanilla extract (1 1/2 tsp.)
- Sour cream (8 oz., low – fat)
- Cinnamon (ground)

Directions:

1. Set a Dutch oven on over high heat with your first 3 ingredients then allow to come to a simmer (about 15 mins).

2. Add salt, and rice, stir and reduce the heat to medium to simmer until tender (about 45 minutes, stirring occasionally).

3. Add your egg to a small bowl than slowly whisk in a cup of your hot rice mixture into it. When fully combined, add back to the Dutch oven.

4. Switch off heat, and stir in your remaining ingredients. Serve, and enjoy.

Chocolate Pudding Pops

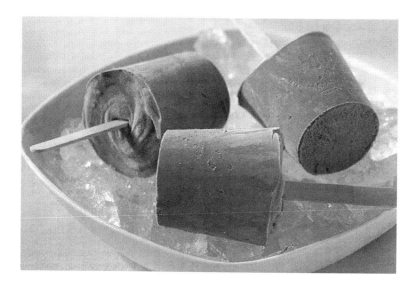

These pudding pops are just as delicious no matter how old you may get.

Serving Size: 6

Overall Time: 4 Hours 15 Mins

Ingredients:

- Milk (2 1/2 cups, 2%)
- Sugar (1/2 cup sugar)
- Cocoa (1/2 cup, unsweetened)
- Cornstarch (1 tbsp.)
- Salt (1/4 tsp.)
- Egg yolk (1 large)
- Vanilla (1 tsp.)
- Chocolate (2 oz., finely chopped)

Directions:

1. Set a medium saucepan over medium heat with your first 6 ingredients, whisk to combine, and allow to cook until bubbly, and thick (about 8 minutes, constantly stirring).

2. Switch off heat, and add chocolate, and vanilla, then stir until smooth.

3. Pour your pudding mixture into an air tight container and place in the center of a bowl filled with ice to cool down.

4. Tightly cover the bowl with plastic wrap, and allow to chill in the refrigerator completely.

5. Transfer your pudding evenly into your ice mop molds, add craft sticks in the center, and set to freeze until set (about 4 hours).

Tart Tangy Bulgur Salad

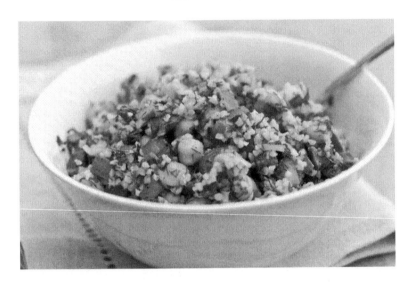

This sweet and tangy salad is bound to stimulate your taste buds.

Serving Size: 4

Overall Time: 1 Hour

Ingredients:

- Bulgur (1 cup, uncooked)
- Boiling water (1 cup)
- Olive oil (2 tbsp.)
- Lime juice (2 tbsp.)
- Salt (1/2 tsp.)
- Basil leaves (8 large, finely chopped)
- Garlic (1 clove, minced)
- Red onion (1/4 cup, chopped)
- Olives (12 large, sliced)
- Tomato (1 large, chopped)

Directions:

1. Add your water and bulgur to a large bowl. Tightly seal, and allow to stand like this for about 45 minutes

2. Add your remaining ingredients, toss to combine, and serve.

Coconut Overnight Oats

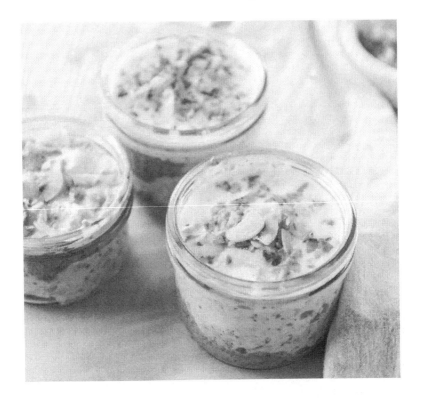

Oats are delicious, filling, and easy to digest.

Yield: 4 Servings

Total Time: 25 Minutes

Ingredients

- 1 cup rolled oats
- 420ml full fat organic coconut milk
- ¼ tsp cinnamon
- ½ tsp wheat germ
- 3 tbsp. chia seeds
- 2 small ripe pears, diced, for serving
- 1 tbsp. pure maple syrup

Directions

1. Combine all the vegan oats ingredients in a medium jar with a lid and stir well to blend all the ingredients together.

2. Cover the jar and chill overnight for the best results.

3. Remove the oats from the fridge and stir well. Enjoy!

Blueberry Ice Cream

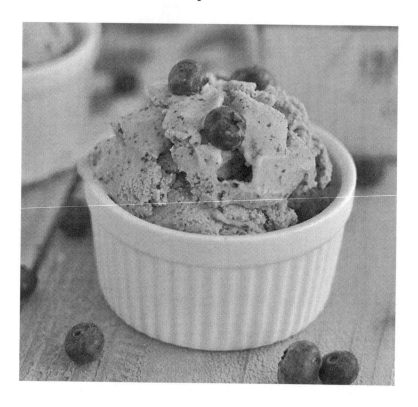

This yummy dessert is perfect for a hot, frustrating chemo day.

Serves: 16

Time: 20 minutes + inactive time

Ingredients:

- 2 cups fresh blueberries
- 1 cup whipping cream
- 4 whole eggs
- 1 cup full-fat milk
- 1 cup filtered water
- ½ cup caster sugar
- 1 teaspoon vanilla paste
- 1 pinches salt

Directions:

1. In a saucepan, whisk the water, milk, eggs, sugar, and salt.

2. Heat the mixture over medium-high heat and bring to a gentle bubble.

3. Strain into a wide bowl and cool.

4. Whisk in the vanilla, whipping cream and fresh blueberries.

5. Cover and chill for 2 hours. Pour the mix into ice cream making machine and process according to manufacturer's instructions.

Tomato Basil Soup

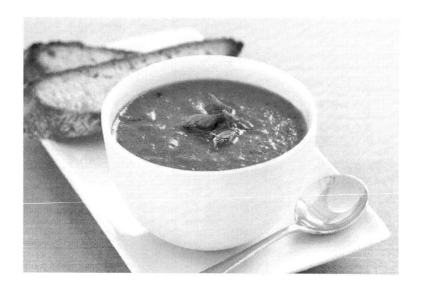

There's nothing that calms the stomach more than a delicious bowl of tomato soup.

Yield: 7 Cups

Total Time: 40 Minutes

Ingredients

- 2 cloves fresh garlic
- 4 cups tomato puree
- 2 cups vegetable broth
- 1/4 cup coconut oil
- 1/2 cup coconut cream
- 1/2 cup fresh basil leaves
- pinch of stevia, if desired
- 1 teaspoon sea salt

Directions

1. Blend together garlic and tomatoes in a blender until very smooth.

2. Pour into your pressure cooker and add broth, coconut oil, and salt.

3. Lock lid and cook on high pressure for 20 minutes.

4. When done, release pressure naturally and then stir in chopped basil and coconut cream.

5. Blend the mixture with an immersion blender until smooth and then serve. Enjoy!

Cream of Butternut Squash Ginger Soup

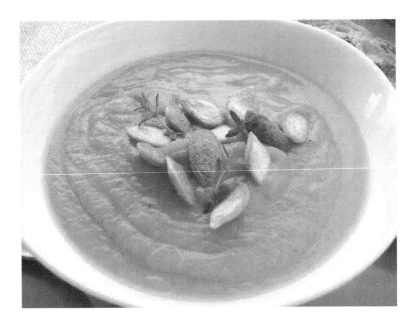

This soup is creamy, and tasty with just enough spice to keep it down.

Yield: 4 Servings

Total Time: 25 Minutes

Ingredients

- 1 teaspoon extra-virgin olive oil
- 1 large onion, roughly chopped
- 1 sprig of Sage
- 4 lb. butternut Squash, diced
- ½" piece of fresh ginger, minced
- ¼ teaspoon nutmeg
- salt and pepper (1/4 tsp. each)
- 4 cups vegetable stock
- ½ cup Toasted Pumpkin Seeds, to serve

Directions

1. In your pressure cooker over medium heat, sauté onion with salt, pepper, and sage until softened.

2. Remove the onion mixture to a bowl and add squash cubes to the pot; sauté for 10 minutes and then add in the remaining ingredients including onion mixture.

3. Lock lid and cook on high pressure for 15 minutes; release pressure naturally and then discard sage.

4. Using an immersion blender, blend the mixture until smooth and serve garnished with toasted salt pumpkin seeds.

Sweet Corn Chicken Noodle Soup

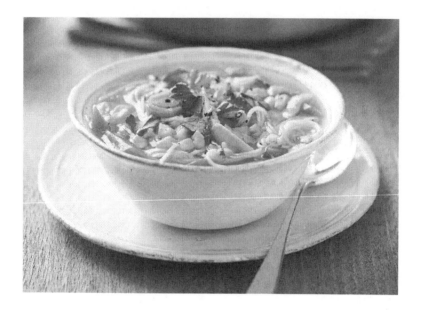

The corn in this recipe adds a nice element of texture, without creating a hazard for digestion.

Serving Size: 4

Overall Time: 1 Hour 1 Minute

Ingredients:

- Chicken Stock (8 cups, fat-free, low-sodium)
- Sweet Corn (8 oz., kernels)
- Chicken breast (12 oz., skinless, boneless, halved)
- Carrots (2 cups, sliced diagonally)
- Celery (2 cups, sliced diagonally)
- Onion (1 cup, chopped)
- Egg noodles (6 oz.)
- Salt (1/2 tsp.)
- Black pepper (1/2 tsp.)

Directions:

1. Set a Dutch oven over medium heat with your first 3 ingredients and allow to come to a boil.

2. Once boiling, reduce heat to low then continue to simmer for about 20 minutes.

3. Set chicken aside, and allow to stand uncovered for 10 minutes. Chop into bite sized pieces, and set aside.

4. Add vegetables, cover, and allow to continue to simmer until fork tender (about 10 minutes) then add noodles, then allow to simmer until fork tender (about 6 minutes).

5. Add in your remaining ingredients, and continue to cook until chicken has been fully heated through. Season to taste and serve.

Tomato Carrot Soup

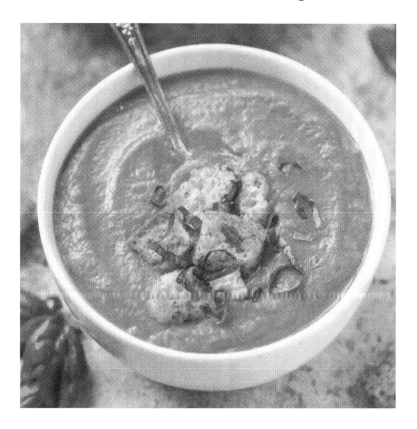

This soup is rich, tasty and nutritious.

Yield: 7 Cups

Total Time: 40 Minutes

Ingredients

- 2 cloves fresh garlic
- 4 cups tomato puree
- 2 cups vegetable broth
- 1/4 cup coconut oil
- 1/2 cup coconut cream
- 1/2 cup fresh chopped carrot
- pinch of sugar, if desired
- 1 teaspoon sea salt

Directions

1. Blend together garlic, carrot, and tomatoes in a blender until very smooth.

2. Pour into your pressure cooker and add broth, coconut oil, and salt.

3. Lock lid and cook on high pressure for 20 minutes.

4. When done, release pressure naturally and then stir in coconut cream.

5. Blend the mixture with an immersion blender until smooth and then serve. Enjoy!

Hearty Vegetable Soup

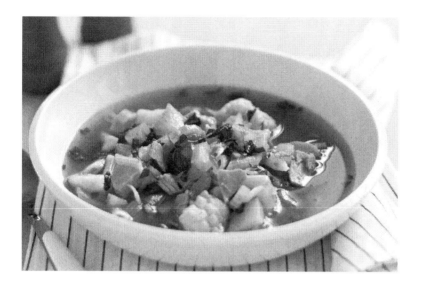

Allow yourself to relax, and enjoy a filling bowl of soup filled with delicious veggies, and packed with flavor.

Yield: 6 Servings

Total Time: 25 Minutes

Ingredients

- 1 tbsp. canola oil
- 1 cup chopped red onion
- 3 organic apples, diced
- 6 cups vegetable broth
- 1/2 tbsp. chopped fresh rosemary
- 1 leek, chopped
- 1/2 tbsp. fresh thyme
- A pinch of cayenne pepper
- A pinch of sea salt

Directions

1. In your pressure cooker over medium heat, add canola oil; stir in onion and sauté for about 4 minutes or until fragrant and golden.

2. Stir in broth and apples and then lock lid; cook on high pressure for 5 minutes and then release pressure naturally.

3. Stir in rosemary, leek, thyme, cayenne pepper, and salt. Serve right away.

Smoked Fish Chowder

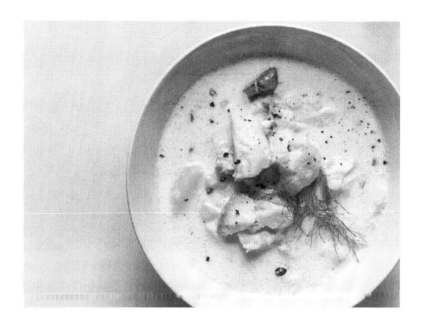

Get a bowl of fishy, delicious goodness with Omega fatty acids in every bite.

Serving Size: 4

Overall Time: 45 Minutes

Ingredients:

- Haddock (1 lb., smoked, fillet)
- Water (1 L.)
- Butter (2 oz.)
- Onions (2, chopped finely)
- Flour (2 tbsp.)
- Potatoes (8 oz., peeled, chopped finely)
- Carrots (6 oz., peeled, chopped finely
- Half and half (140ml)
- Salt and black pepper (1/4 tsp.)

Directions:

1. Set your water on in a large saucepan and allow to come to boil.

2. Reduce your heat to low and add your haddock. Allow to cook until tender (about 10 minutes).

3. Remove haddock from stock, flake and set aside then discard bones, and skin.

4. In a separate saucepan, add butter, and set over medium heat.

5. Once melted, add onions and cook, while stirring, until soft. Next, add flour and cook, while stirring, to create what's called a roux (about a minute).

6. Stir in your fish water (stock) gradually and allow to return to a boil.

7. Add in your remaining ingredients, except haddock and cream, then allow to cook on a simmer until veggies are fork tender (about 10 minutes).

8. Add fish and half and half cream. Season to taste and serve.

Lazy Lentil Stew

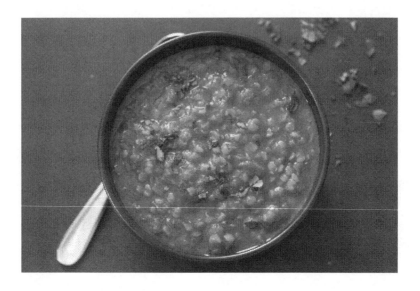

Lentils in this recipe are used to provide nutritious content, as well as, texture in every spoon of soup.

Yield: 4-6 Servings

Total Time: 20 Minutes

Ingredients

- ½ cup dry navy beans
- ½ cup dry red lentils
- 5 small carrots, sliced
- 1 cup barley
- ½ cup red wine
- 900 ml vegetable juice
- 2 cups celery, sliced
- ¼ cup brown sugar
- 2 large onions, chopped
- 2 bay leaves
- 1 tsp. freshly ground black pepper
- ½ tsp. thyme
- A good pinch garlic powder
- ¼ salt to taste
- 2 cups water

Directions

1. Combine all the ingredients in your pressure cooker and lock lid.

2. Cook on high pressure for 10 minutes.

3. Release the pressure naturally and then discard the bay leaves before serving.

4. Enjoy!

Easy Red Onion Apple Soup

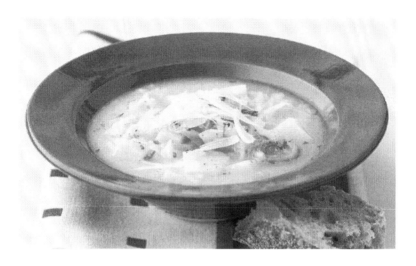

Yield: 6 Servings

Total Time: 25 Minutes

Ingredients

- 1 tbsp. canola oil
- 1 cup chopped red onion
- 3 organic apples, diced
- 8 cups vegetable broth
- 1/2 tbsp. chopped fresh rosemary
- 1 leek, chopped
- 1/2 tbsp. fresh thyme
- A pinch of cayenne pepper
- A pinch of sea salt

Directions

1. In a medium saucepan, heat canola oil; stir in onion and sauté for about 4 minutes or until fragrant and golden.

2. Transfer the sautéed onion to your pressure cooker over medium heat, and stir in broth and bring the mixture to a gentle boil.

3. Stir in the apples, leek, thyme and rosemary and lock lid. Cook on high pressure for 10 minutes.

4. When done, release pressure naturally and then season with salt and pepper and serve.

Bean Dip

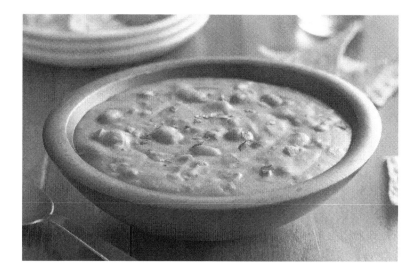

This dip is an amazing dip to pair with your favorite cracker for a late afternoon snack.

Serving Size: 3

Overall Time: 20 Minutes

Ingredients:

- Butter Beans (14 oz.)
- Lemon (1, grated and juiced)
- Tahini (1 tbsp.)
- Olive oil (1 tbsp.)
- Garlic (1 clove, crushed)
- Salt and black pepper (1/4 tsp., each)

Directions:

1. Drain, and rinse beans, then set aside to drain.

2. Add bean to a food processor, and process until smooth.

3. Transfer your bean paste to a small mixing bowl, then add in your remaining ingredients.

4. Stir to combine, and serve with your favorite cracker.

One-Pot Fish with Black Olives Tomatoes

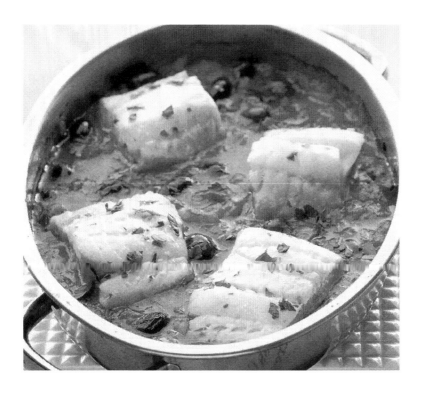

This delicious combo is nutrient dense, tasty and just melts in your mouth.

Serving Size: 4

Overall Time: 35 Minutes

Ingredients:

- Black olives (6 oz., with oil, stones discarded)
- Onion (1 large, chopped roughly)
- Tomatoes (14 oz., chopped)
- Cod (24 oz., boneless, fillets)
- Salt and black pepper (1 tsp. each)
- Parsley (1 tbsp, chopped)
- Lemon (4 wedges)

Directions:

1. Set oven to preheat to 400 degrees F.

2. Set am ovenproof saucepan with a tablespoon of oil from olives over medium heat until hot.

3. Add onion and cook, while stirring, until soft.

4. Add tomatoes and season with salt, and pepper.

5. Allow to come to a boil, then add olives.

6. Add fish skin side down in sauce. Spoon a splash of the olive oil over the fish.

7. Set to bake, without cover, until the fish is fully cooked (about 15 minutes).sh is cooked.

8. Season to taste, top with parsley, and lemon wedges. Serve.

Chicken Thighs with Crumbed Tomatoes

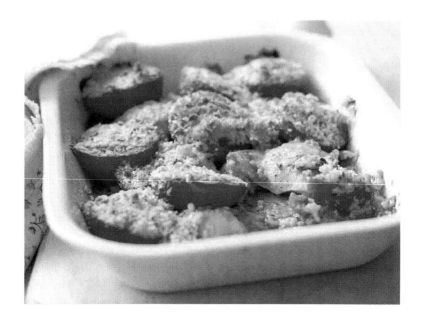

Here is another deliciously healthy dinner you can enjoy at any night of the week.

Serving Size: 6

Overall Time: 1 Hour

Ingredients:

- Chicken thighs (6)
- Breadcrumbs (2 oz.)
- Chicken stock (150ml)
- Olive oil (1 tbsp.)
- Tomatoes (6, halved)
- Fresh oregano (1 tbsp., chopped)
- Parmesan cheese (2 tbsp., grated)

Directions:

1. Set oven to preheat to 350 degrees F. Season chicken to taste with salt, and pepper.

2. Set a skillet with oil over medium heat to get hot.

3. Add onions then cook, while stirring, until soft.

4. Add chicken thighs and cook until golden on both sides.

5. Remove from skillet and drain excess oil with paper towel. Set drained chicken in a lightly greased baking dish.

6. Set a tomato half on top of chicken thigh then top evenly with remaining seasoning.

7. Add stock around chicken, and set to bake until fully cooked through (about 45 minutes).

8. Serve, and enjoy.

Black Bean Chipotle Soup

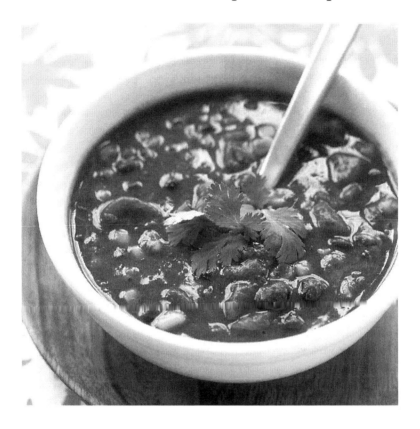

This soup is easy to make and unbelievably delicious.

Yield: 6 servings

Total Time: 28 Minutes

Ingredients:

- 1 tbsp. extra virgin olive oil
- 2 medium red onions, diced
- 1 red bell pepper, diced
- 1 green bell pepper, diced
- 4 tsp. ground cumin
- 4 garlic cloves, minced
- 16 ounces dried black beans
- 7 cups hot water
- 1 tbsp. chopped chipotle chilies
- 2 tsp. coarse kosher salt
- 2 tsp. fresh lime juice
- 1/4 tsp. ground black pepper

Directions:

1. In a large skillet set over medium high heat, heat olive oil until hot but not smoky.

2. Sauté bell peppers and onion for about 8 minutes or until brown.

3. Stir in cumin and garlic for about 1 minute, transfer the mixture to your pressure cooker.

4. Stir in add 7 cups water, chipotles and beans and lock lid.

5. Cook on high pressure for 10 minutes and the release the pressure naturally.

6. Transfer about 4 cups of the mixture to a blender and blend until very smooth

7. Return the puree to the pot and stir in salt, lime juice, and pepper until well combined.

8. Ladle the soup into serving bowls and top with coconut cream and avocado.

Split Pea Soup w/ Navy Beans Sweet Potatoes

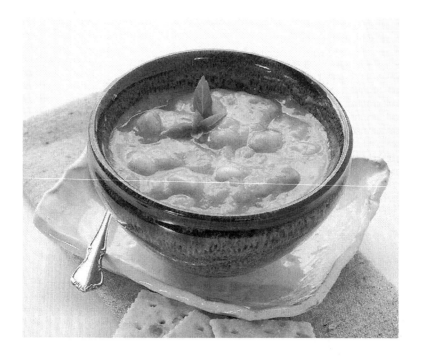

Here is yet another easy bean soup that will provide you with adequate nutrients while allow your body to easily digest it.

Yield: 4-6 Servings

Total Time: 40 Minutes

Ingredients

- ½ cup dried navy beans
- 1 cup split peas
- 1 medium sweet potato, diced
- 1/2 cup nutritional yeast
- ½ teaspoon liquid smoke
- 2 bay leaves
- Pinch of pepper
- Pinch of sea salt
- 5 cups water

Directions

1. In a pressure cooker, mix navy beans, split peas, sweet potatoes, water and liquid smoke.

2. Cook on high pressure for 20 minutes.

3. Natural release pressure and stir in salt, pepper, and nutritional yeast. Serve.

Tuna Vegetable Spaghetti

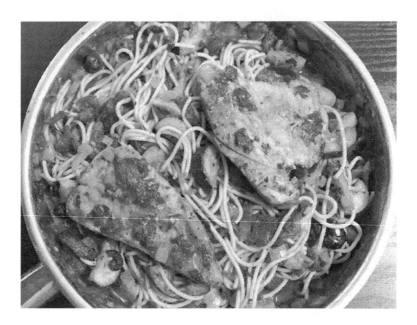

This delicious meal is filling, tasty, and can be enjoyed by your family.

Serving Size: 4

Overall Time: 17 Minutes

Ingredients:

- Spaghetti (10 oz., dried)
- Mixed vegetable (14 oz., frozen)
- Lasagna sauce (18 oz., white)
- Tuna (7 oz., each, drained)

Directions:

1. Set your spaghetti to boil in a large saucepan (about 5-6 minutes). Add mixed vegetables and continue to cook for another 5 minutes. Then drain and set aside.

2. Add your lasagna sauce, and tuna into the now empty saucepan, and return to heat for another minute.

3. Return the remaining ingredients to the saucepan, stir, and continue cooking until fully heated through. Season with salt, and pepper.

Quick Shepherd's Pie

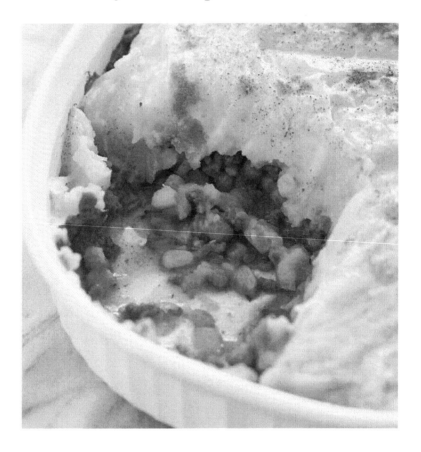

Enjoy a small taste of Britain with this delicious Sheppard's pie, fit for the whole family.

Serving Size: 4

Overall Time: 40 Minutes

Ingredients:

- Onion (1, diced)
- Carrots (2, diced)
- Worcestershire sauce (2 tbsp.)
- Rosemary (1 tsp., dried)
- Onion gravy granules (2 tbsp.)
- Olive oil (1 tbsp.)
- Baguettes (2, garlic, frozen, sliced)
- Frozen peas (3 oz.)

Directions:

1. Set your oven to preheat to 400 degrees F.

2. Set a large saucepan with oil over medium heat to get hot.

3. Add rosemary, carrots, onion, and lamb mince and cook, while stirring for 5 minutes.

4. Add peas, Worcestershire sauce, peas, water, and gravy granules.

5. Allow to simmer, covered while stirring occasionally for about 10 minutes.

6. Transfer your mixture into lightly greased glass baking dish.

7. Top with garlic baguette slices then lightly drizzle with a bit of olive oil.

8. Set to bake until golden brown (about 15 minutes).

Conclusion

We are elated that you were able to complete all 30 healthy delicious recipes to enjoy during chemo therapy. The next step from here is to continue practicing until you have perfected each one. After that, you can always find another amazing journey to partake in from cuisines across the globe in another one of our books. We hope to see you again soon. Happy cooking!

Author's Afterthoughts

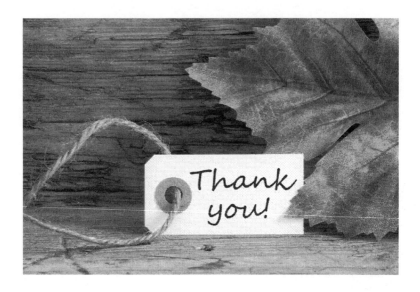

Thanks ever so much to each of my cherished readers for investing the time to read this book!

I know you could have picked from many other books but you chose this one. So a big thanks for downloading this book and reading all the way to the end.

If you enjoyed this book or received value from it, I'd like to ask you for a favor. Please take a few minutes to post an honest and heartfelt review on Amazon.com. Your support does make a difference and helps to benefit other people.

Thanks!

Daniel Humphreys

About the Author

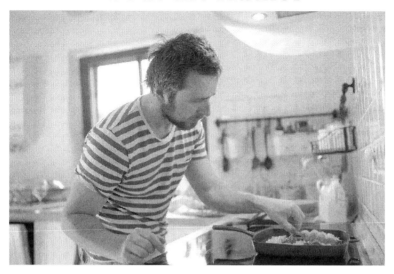

Daniel Humphreys

Many people will ask me if I am German or Norman, and my answer is that I am 100% unique! Joking aside, I owe my cooking influence mainly to my mother who was British! I can certainly make a mean Sheppard's pie, but when it comes to preparing Bratwurst sausages and drinking beer with friends, I am also all in!

I am taking you on this culinary journey with me and hope you can appreciate my diversified background. In my 15 years career as a chef, I never had a dish returned to me by one of clients, so that should say something about me! Actually, I will take that back. My worst critic is my four years old son, who refuses to taste anything that is green color. That shall pass, I am sure.

My hope is to help my children discover the joy of cooking and sharing their creations with their loved ones, like I did all my life. When you develop a passion for cooking and my suspicious is that you have one as well, it usually sticks for life. The best advice I can give anyone as a professional chef is invest. Invest your time, your heart in each meal you are creating. Invest also a little money in good cooking hardware and quality ingredients. But most of all enjoy every meal you prepare with YOUR friends and family!

Made in the
USA
Middletown, DE